Tuberculosis—A Complex Health Threat

A Policy Primer of Global TB Challenges

Authors
Phillip Nieburg
Talia Dubovi
Sahil Angelo

A Report of the CSIS Global Health Policy Center

April 2015

CSIS | CENTER FOR STRATEGIC &
INTERNATIONAL STUDIES

ROWMAN &
LITTLEFIELD

Lanham • Boulder • New York • London

About CSIS

For over 50 years, the Center for Strategic and International Studies (CSIS) has worked to develop solutions to the world's greatest policy challenges. Today, CSIS scholars are providing strategic insights and bipartisan policy solutions to help decisionmakers chart a course toward a better world.

CSIS is a nonprofit organization headquartered in Washington, D.C. The Center's 220 full-time staff and large network of affiliated scholars conduct research and analysis and develop policy initiatives that look into the future and anticipate change.

Founded at the height of the Cold War by David M. Abshire and Admiral Arleigh Burke, CSIS was dedicated to finding ways to sustain American prominence and prosperity as a force for good in the world. Since 1962, CSIS has become one of the world's preeminent international institutions focused on defense and security; regional stability; and transnational challenges ranging from energy and climate to global health and economic integration.

Former U.S. senator Sam Nunn has chaired the CSIS Board of Trustees since 1999. Former deputy secretary of defense John J. Hamre became the Center's president and chief executive officer in 2000.

CSIS does not take specific policy positions; accordingly, all views expressed herein should be understood to be solely those of the author(s).

Acknowledgments

This report is made possible by the generous support of the Bill & Melinda Gates Foundation.

ISBN: 978-1-4422-4094-0 (pb); 978-1-4422-4095-7 (eBook)

Center for Strategic & International Studies
1616 Rhode Island Avenue, NW
Washington, DC 20036
202-887-0200 | www.csis.org

Rowman & Littlefield
4501 Forbes Boulevard
Lanham, MD 20706
301-459-3366 | www.rowman.com

| Contents

| Preface

The pervasiveness of global tuberculosis (TB) poses a particular set of challenges to policymakers. In order to make the necessary strategic decisions, it is essential to understand how the disease works and its impact on individuals, families, communities, and broader global health goals. This primer is intended to lay out the basics for a nontechnical audience to give policymakers the information they need to make informed and accurate decisions about the future of U.S. TB control efforts. The Executive Summary highlights the key points and main takeaways; the subsequent primer addresses these issues in more detail.

| Executive Summary

Tuberculosis, or TB, is one of the oldest ailments in recorded human history and remains one of the deadliest. In 2013, TB claimed the lives of 1.5 million people worldwide, making it second only to HIV/AIDS as the leading infectious killer of adults globally.

Over the last several decades, a concerted international effort to control TB has made significant progress, with prevalence and mortality rates dropping by 41 percent and 45 percent, respectively, since the early 1990s. Improved screening and testing methods, enhanced surveillance and contact tracing, greater access to effective drugs, and better monitoring of treatment protocols have saved millions of lives and reduced the burden of TB throughout the world.

And yet, it is not nearly enough. The year 2013 saw 9 million new cases, which in addition to death and disability lead to staggering economic costs, both at the individual and systemic levels. One-third of cases are unreported—either undiagnosed or treated with unknown standards in private health systems—which significantly hampers efforts to reduce the spread of disease. Rising drug resistance threatens recent progress as well as dramatically increases the cost of treatment. TB's complex biology and epidemiology means that its ongoing prevalence also impacts global efforts against HIV/AIDS, diabetes, and other important health challenges.

TB is biologically complex, which complicates TB control efforts. TB is an airborne bacterial disease that is mainly transmitted from person-to-person. Primarily impacting the lungs, TB causes chronic cough, fever, night sweats, bloody sputum, and/or weight loss, and over half of patients with untreated TB will die. Those who survive are often incapacitated for weeks or months, and many are left with permanently reduced lung capacity.

Treatment regimens for TB require daily administration of multiple drugs for six to nine months. The length of treatment is necessary to fully eliminate the disease, but adherence to the full treatment regime is challenging as patients often begin to feel better within a matter of days or weeks and do not follow through with the complete treatment. Because a failure to complete the full course of drugs can lead to the development of drug-resistant TB, ensuring that patients finish their entire treatment is both a priority and a challenge for TB control programs.

TB can also lie dormant in an individual, walled off by the body's immune system. Known as latent TB infection, the bacteria can live in an individual for his or her entire life and never become active TB disease—in fact, only approximately 10 percent of people with latent TB will eventually develop the active disease. People with latent TB are neither symptomatic nor contagious. The exact biological causes of TB activation are not fully known, but activation often occurs in people with suppressed immune response, including infants, the elderly, and those with certain diseases such as HIV/AIDS, diabetes, and some types of cancers. Prophylactic treatment of latent infection can reduce, but not eliminate, the chances that the disease will activate and is recommended for certain high-risk groups, such as people in high TB burden areas or people living with HIV. Roughly one-third of the world's population has latent TB.

TB screening tests can determine the presence of TB infection but cannot distinguish between latent and active disease, meaning a longer and much more costly diagnosis process is necessary to distinguish between those who need immediate treatment and those who may not. New technology, such as GeneXpert, can reduce the time required for a definitive diagnosis but is expensive (in terms of initial investment as well as operational costs) and inaccessible to much of the world. The development of faster, less expensive, and portable diagnostic tools could have a significant impact on efforts to identify and treat TB patients.

The emergence of drug-resistant TB increases the costs of all TB control programs. Drug resistance develops when the bacteria infecting an individual evolve to a point where one or more TB drugs become ineffective at treating that person's disease. While resistance develops in individuals, it can be spread from person to person. Resistance ranges from *mono-resistant TB* that is resistant to a single TB drug, to *multidrug-resistant TB* (MDR-TB) that is resistant to at least two of the most commonly used and least expensive TB drugs, to *extensively resistant TB* (XDR-TB) that is resistant to at least two "first line" drugs as well as at least two of the "second line" alternative treatments.

Treatment of drug-resistant TB is longer and significantly more expensive, with more severe adverse effects on the patient and higher death rates. While currently only an estimated 5 percent of global TB cases are drug resistant, the existence of resistant strains increases the costs of screening and diagnosis for all patients, since every individual must be assessed for resistance patterns in order to appropriately select an effective treatment. In order to avoid the development of resistance, all patients with drug-sensitive TB must complete their full course of treatment, which requires significant investment by health workers to ensure full compliance. The adverse effects of second line TB drugs—which are likely more severe in low- and middle-income countries that do not have access to the full range of treatment options—further reduces patient adherence to treatment protocols and in turn increases the opportunities for additional resistance to develop. The development of shorter treatment regimens for both drug-sensitive and drug-resistant TB would be a major step toward reducing the impact of drug resistance.

TB interacts with other diseases—most notably HIV/AIDS and diabetes. TB and HIV are linked: in people infected with both, each disease increases the severity and accelerates the course of the illness of the other. TB remains the single most common cause of death of people living with HIV, responsible for at least 25 percent of 1.5 million global AIDS deaths in 2013. Conversely, approximately 25 percent of TB deaths occurred in people living with HIV, and progression from latent to active TB is 25–50 times more likely in those infected with HIV.

The connection between TB and HIV/AIDS means that in areas of high burden of both diseases, programs aimed at preventing and treating one of these diseases must also address the other. Patients should be tested for both diseases and TB and HIV programs must coordinate at the local, national, and international levels. While some efforts are being made to better address TB/HIV coinfection, the lack of sufficient attention to the connection between the diseases threatens the long-term success of major HIV/AIDS initiatives, most notably the President's Emergency Plan for AIDS Relief (PEPFAR).

Diabetes also interacts with TB. Progression from latent to active TB is three times higher in patients with diabetes, and diabetics are five times more likely to develop MDR-TB. In addition, the symptoms of TB in people with both diseases differ from traditional TB symptoms, making detection more difficult and increasing the misdiagnosis rate. There is evidence that TB and diabetes drugs may counteract each other, further complicating the picture.

Global diabetes rates are predicted to double in the next 15 years. Eighty percent of this predicted future burden will be in developing countries, where at least one-third of the population has latent TB. The confluence of these two diseases means more attention to the connection between diabetes and TB will be necessary to prevent the growing burden of diabetes from also causing an analogous spike in TB.

The costs of TB are devastating for individuals and families, as well as health systems. TB is fundamentally a disease of poverty. It disproportionately affects the poor, in part because of the risk factors associated with poverty that increase susceptibility to TB: poor ventilation, overcrowded living and working conditions, malnutrition, and lack of access to health systems for diagnosis and treatment. TB also perpetuates poverty: the family of the average TB patient loses more than 50 percent of its annual income to direct health costs, transportation costs, and lost income from forgone work.

TB is also costly for health systems. The per patient cost of treating TB varies by location and drug resistance patterns, but the cost to treat drug-sensitive TB in most high burden countries ranges from $100 to $500 per patient, while the average cost of treating MDR-TB ranges from $10,000 per patient in low-income countries to over $130,000 per patient in higher-income countries like the United States. The economic impact on individuals also reaches the broader economy, through the cumulative impact of lost income and missed work, particularly in high burden areas.

More focus on TB is needed. The bottom line is that TB is highly expensive and debilitating, with the potential for catastrophic health and financial impacts for individuals, families, and health systems. Globally, funding available for TB control efforts is at least $2 billion short of what is needed to properly address the disease burden, not including the funding needed for research and development. There are many opportunities for the global community to act to dramatically improve outcomes, from developing better screening methods, diagnostic tools, and treatment options to improving coordination between TB efforts and others major global health initiatives to creating new financing options and improved supply chains for drugs. Without greater effort, this ancient disease will continue to be a major global burden for years to come.

| Introduction

Tuberculosis, or TB, is one of the oldest diseases in recorded human history and remains one of the deadliest. In 2013, TB claimed the lives of 1.5 million people worldwide,[1] making it second only to HIV/AIDS as the leading infectious killer of adults.

Globally, an estimated 11 million people were living with active TB in 2013,[2] of which 9 million cases newly occurred that year.[3] Southeast Asian and Western Pacific countries accounted for nearly 60 percent of new TB cases, with just under 30 percent in Africa. Approximately 3.3 million (37 percent) of the 9 million new cases occurred in women and about 550,000 in children. HIV is also an important contributor to the global burden of TB; an estimated 1.1 million of the new TB cases occurred in people living with HIV (PLHIV), and TB/HIV coinfection accounted for 25 percent of the 1.5 million TB deaths that year.

The 9 million new TB cases occurring in 2013 included the actual 5.7 million cases reported through national TB programs plus an estimated 3 million "missed cases" that went unreported. Some of these missed cases were in people who were sick with symptoms of TB but who did not seek care; others were in people who received health care but were not diagnosed with TB. A final missed group was those people diagnosed with TB in the nongovernmental health sector but were not reported to national TB surveillance systems. The quality of TB care and treatment provided to this latter group is unknown.

In addition to the death and physical disability caused by global TB, its direct and indirect economic costs have been—and remain—staggering. The family of the average TB patient loses more than 50 percent of its annual income to direct health costs, transportation costs, and lost income from foregone work; up to 50 percent of TB-affected families sell household items to help pay for care during the months and sometimes years required for successful treatment.[4]

Beyond the health and economic burdens linked to traditional drug-sensitive TB, drug-resistant TB bacteria have emerged, requiring longer courses of treatment with alternative drug regimens that are not only far less effective but also compromised by severe adverse effects that can include depression and deafness. These treatment

---

[1] World Health Organization, *Global Tuberculosis Report 2014* (Geneva: WHO, October 2014), xi. http://www.who.int/tb/publications/global_report/en/.
[2] Ibid., 19.
[3] Ibid., 7.
[4] World Health Organization, "Eliminating the financial hardship of TB via Universal Health Coverage and Other Social Protection Measures," 2013, http://www.who.int/tb/publications/UHC_SP_factsheet.pdf.

regimens are also expensive and often in short supply. In addition to drug resistance, TB is further complicated by its interactions with other diseases such as HIV and diabetes.

Over the last several decades, concerted global TB-control efforts have had an important impact, with overall TB disease and mortality rates dropping by 41 percent and 45 percent, respectively, since the early 1990s. Between 2000 and 2013, a combination of improved screening and testing methods, enhanced surveillance and contact tracing, greater access to effective TB drugs, and direct observation of treatment (DOT) reduced the burden of TB throughout the world and are estimated to have saved 37 million lives.[5]

Unfortunately, these efforts are not nearly enough. The global TB burden persists, and there remain major gaps in TB-control efforts. For example, only 48 percent of persons with multidrug-resistant TB were successfully treated in 2011,[6] resulting in ongoing disease transmission from the others. More broadly, the continuing transmission of drug-sensitive and drug-resistant TB poses a significant global health challenge, including to the United States and other industrialized countries.

For years, policymakers, health workers, and others who work on global TB have been calling on the international community to do more: more support for overall strengthening of national TB programs; more and better screening, testing, and case notification to uncover the millions of undiagnosed and unreported cases; more research to discover and develop more effective and less onerous treatment regimens, including for drug-resistant TB; more and better prophylaxis for those with latent TB infections to prevent the development of active TB disease[7]; and above all, more resources to support these efforts.

Those resources have not materialized, and there is little current evidence to suggest that they will appear in the foreseeable future. The overall U.S. global health budget has flat-lined, recent budget proposals from the U.S. administration have been consistent in calling for budget cuts for global TB, and globally, few new donors or other new funding sources are on the horizon.

It is therefore essential that policymakers direct those limited TB resources to where they will have the most impact. Because evidence suggests that TB interventions in specific populations and specific hot spots could significantly stem the spread of disease, global TB-control efforts must become even more strategic and targeted, focusing on areas of greatest impact.

---

[5] World Health Organization, *Global Tuberculosis Report 2014*, xi.
[6] Ibid., 68.
[7] Latent TB infection will be discussed later in this report.

TB infection and disease are biologically complicated, and effective TB control is influenced by economic, cultural, social, and political factors in every society it touches. Global TB-control efforts involve a wide array of actors, including several U.S. government agencies, each with its own area of responsibility in global TB-control efforts. Charting the best overall course forward will require the ability to navigate myriad complexities and competing priorities and U.S. and international decisionmakers must understand the basics of TB infection, TB disease, and TB control in order to make optimal policy and budgetary decisions.

To that end, we provide a primer of the most critical factors about the spread and burden of TB and the critical issues involved in successful programs for its control.

1 | The Epidemiology, Pathology, and Biology of Tuberculosis

TB is an airborne disease caused by *Mycobacterium tuberculosis* bacteria that are primarily spread from person to person. When someone with active TB disease in his or her lung(s) or throat coughs or sneezes, or even yells or sings, droplets containing TB bacteria can be spread into the air.[8] These TB-laden droplets can remain airborne in still air (e.g., inside closed rooms) for several hours, meaning that transmission of TB to a new human host does not have to be immediate. When breathed in by others, these bacteria-laden droplets can reach the lung sacs (alveoli), where a new TB infection can begin. Such airborne spread of TB infection to others is most likely to occur with close contacts such as family members, friends, or in school or work.

TB is primarily a lung (pulmonary) disease.[9] People with pulmonary TB can have symptoms of chronic cough, fever, night sweats, bloody sputum (phlegm), and/or weight loss. By definition, TB is considered a chronic disease because it lasts more than a month; TB disease in untreated individuals typically last for two to three years, during which there is ongoing transmission to family and community members. Over half of untreated TB patients die of their disease while others enter periods of remission and relapse that may last decades. Patients whose TB disease is identified and treated in a timely manner will be isolated for several weeks, until their TB is confirmed to no longer be contagious. Even after that, it may be a few months until patients feel well enough to resume their normal activities. Furthermore, many TB survivors have permanently reduced breathing capacity due to scar tissue in their lung(s). Sometimes, in patients with complex forms of TB, one or more lobes (sections) of lung have to be surgically removed, causing even greater reductions in lung capacity.[10]

TB bacteria multiply and grow much more slowly than nearly all other bacteria and far slower than viruses such as influenza, measles, or Ebola. The longer bacterial growth cycles characteristic of slow growth means that both TB diagnosis and TB treatment require more time than for nearly all other infections. The slow bacterial

---

[8] Institute of Medicine, *Ending Neglect: The Elimination of Tuberculosis in the United States* (Washington, DC: National Academies Press 2000), 15, http://www.cdc.gov/niosh/nas/rdrp/appendices/chapter6/a6-5.pdf.
[9] TB disease can also occur in organs outside the lungs such as bone, kidney, and brain. Such *extra-pulmonary* TB disease is found more often in people with suppressed immune systems, including young children, people living with HIV or cancer, and people taking immunosuppressive drugs to treat other illnesses. Some patients can have TB simultaneously in their lung(s) and one or more other organ(s).
[10] It has been estimated that TB survivors in the United States lose an average of more than three years of life expectancy. S. Hoger et al., "Longevity loss among cured tuberculosis patients and the potential value of prevention," *International Journal of Tuberculosis and Lung Disease* 18, no. 11 (2014): 1347–52.

growth explains why development of quick diagnostic tools has been elusive. (Treatment and diagnosis are addressed in more detail, below.)

Latent TB Infection

In some cases, particularly in persons with weakened immune systems, an initial TB infection leads quickly to *active TB disease*, with the symptoms described above, the ability to transmit TB infection to others, and all the risks—including death—associated with TB. However, in most circumstances, the body's immune system initially can contain and wall off the TB bacteria, preventing or delaying progression to active TB disease. People with these walled-off TB bacteria have a *latent TB infection*: they do not feel sick and cannot spread TB to others, but TB bacteria are still alive in their bodies. Roughly one-third of the world's population—including approximately 11 million people in the United States—has latent TB infection.[11]

Although latent TB infection can progress to active TB disease at any point after the original infection, it can also remain quiescent for life in many people, meaning they will never develop active TB disease. The lifetime risk of activation for most people with latent TB is only 5 to 10 percent. The exact triggers for progression to active disease are not fully understood; however, certain risk factors are known. The chance of progression is much higher—as high as 10 percent every year—among people who have a suppressed immune response, including young children, persons taking immunosuppressive drugs (e.g., for psoriasis or rheumatoid arthritis), and persons with diabetes, HIV/AIDS, or certain types of cancers.

The overall risk of progression from latent TB infection to active TB disease can be greatly reduced—although not totally eliminated—by any of several drug treatment regimens. (Prevention of TB disease is discussed in more detail below.)

---

[11] Diane Bennett et al., "Prevalence of tuberculosis infection in the United States population: The National Health and Nutrition Survey, 1999–2000," *American Journal of Respiratory and Critical Care Medicine* 177 (2008): 348–55.

2 | Screening and Testing for TB Infection and TB Disease

The methods used to identify people with latent TB infection and active TB disease vary in sophistication, cost, accuracy, and availability. *Screening for TB infection* and *diagnosing TB disease* are two separate but related concepts.

Screening for TB Infection

The TB screening process looks for evidence of the presence of TB infection, although screening tests may not be able to differentiate clearly between a latent TB infection and active TB disease. Thus, while TB screening is an important tool to identify those who have been infected with TB, a positive TB screening test should be followed by additional diagnostic procedures to assess whether the TB is in the form of latent infection or active disease.

The most common TB screening process used in the United States and many other countries begins with a TB skin test, which requires injecting a small amount of inactivated TB extract (tuberculin) just under the skin. In most people whose immune systems have previously responded to a TB infection, the skin test site will redden and swell slightly within 48–72 hours. When the patient returns after that time, the size of any area of redness and swelling will provide a rough clue to the existence of TB infection.[12] Although "false-negative" skin test responses can occur occasionally in persons with suppressed immune systems, no redness or swelling at 48–72 hours generally means no TB infection.[13] An increasingly common alternative to the skin test is a TB blood test that identifies the presence of a chemical in the blood that is produced by the immune system after it has been in contact with TB bacteria or other mycobacteria of the same bacterial family.

---

[12] The TB skin test is often slightly positive (i.e., slightly inflamed or swollen) in people who had been vaccinated with BCG (Bacillus Calmétte-Guérin), a TB vaccine not used in the United States because of the low risk of TB infection and because of its uncertain efficacy in preventing TB disease. BCG vaccine is routinely given to newborns at birth in many low- or middle-income countries. However, while TB infections usually cause a larger and more inflamed tuberculin skin test (TST) response than those due to BCG, a TB blood test is still required to exclude positive skin tests due to BCG vaccine.

[13] If these initial screening skin test or blood tests are negative, then the patient most likely does not have a TB infection. Sometimes, however, patients whose TB infection occurred many years ago may have a false negative skin reaction because their TB immunity has waned and their immune system does not react strongly to a first skin test. However, that first skin test is likely to boost the immune system and, if TB is strongly suspected, a second skin may be "positive" if done several weeks later. In addition, because TB screening tests may not become positive until 8–10 weeks after a TB infection first occurs, any patient with *very recent* exposure *to* TB may need to return for another skin test once that 8- to 10-week period has passed.

Because most current TB skin tests and TB blood tests cannot reliably distinguish between latent TB infection and active TB disease, any "positive" TB screening test should be followed by a second phase of screening. This second screening phase usually involves a chest X-ray to look for evidence of past or current pulmonary (lung) TB. If the chest X-ray result shows no findings consistent with active TB disease and the patient has no symptoms of TB in other organs, then the patient probably has a latent TB infection. If, on the other hand, the chest X-ray is "positive," indicating the possibility of TB lung disease, then specific TB diagnostic testing is required.

In some busy high-risk settings, such as HIV/AIDS clinics in developing countries, initial TB screening can be four simple questions, asking patients whether they have had: (1) a cough for three or more weeks, (2) recent fever, (3) recent "night sweats," or (4) recent weight loss. These questions can identify people who *might* have TB disease and who therefore need more detailed screening with a skin test, chest X-ray, and/or specific diagnostic testing.

Testing for a Specific Diagnosis of TB Disease

In contrast to TB screening, TB diagnostic testing seeks to determine whether an existing TB infection identified through screening is a latent infection or active TB disease. In addition, patients with signs or symptoms of TB disease may require diagnostic testing even in the absence of a positive TB skin or blood test. Compared to TB screening methods, methods for confirming a diagnosis of TB disease may require greater technical skill, are often more costly, and, for some, require additional time for results to become available.

The most common TB diagnostic test begins with an examination under a microscope of sputum (phlegm, *not* just saliva) coughed up by the patient. With the use of special chemical stains, experienced technicians can reliably and quickly (within an hour) identify TB bacteria in the sputum of many—but not all—patients who have active TB lung disease. Depending on the sophistication of the health system, specimens of that same sputum can be sent to a laboratory to see if TB bacteria will grow when kept in an incubator over several weeks. Although this culture testing takes much longer due to TB's extremely slow growth rate, a laboratory culture of live TB bacteria remains the gold standard for identifying TB disease. (In some patients with active TB disease, the culture will grow TB bacteria even if the sputum test under the microscope was negative.)

The recent advent of molecular testing machines, such as GeneXpert, has addressed some of the challenges of sputum culture. These systems can confirm active TB disease by identifying the presence of TB bacterial DNA.[14] They are fast, require limited technical expertise, and can differentiate between drug-sensitive and drug-

---

[14] The GeneXpert and other DNA-based tests will *not* identify patients with latent tuberculosis infection.

resistant TB infections (although they cannot yet identify the specific drug-resistance pattern that determines the necessary drug treatment regimen). These systems also require a very large initial expense for the hardware as well as ongoing access to electricity, and, for GeneXpert, a nearly $10 outlay to pay for the testing cartridge for each individual patient. In addition, recent research on patient outcomes indicates that, as with other TB diagnostic methods, the economic and disease benefits of GeneXpert and similar tests depend heavily on whether patients adhere to the follow-up recommendations and how often health care providers refer patients to public-sector clinics.

3 | Treatment of Active TB Disease

The first successful TB drug, streptomycin, was discovered in 1943 and its value for treating TB disease was well documented by the late 1940s. Other TB drugs were developed soon thereafter. However, it quickly became clear that use of only a single TB drug in a patient led to bacterial resistance to that drug; TB treatment regimens using multiple drugs rapidly became the norm as a way of forestalling development of drug resistance.

Currently, the four "first-line" TB drugs used to treat drug-sensitive TB are now available in most countries and are used in a standard regimen that was developed in the 1970s. This regimen usually requires daily administration of four different drugs for the first few months followed by a continuation of two of these drugs for a total treatment period of six to nine months.

 The months-long duration of such standard TB treatment poses a particular challenge for both patients and TB programs. The regimen frequently has side effects and many patients who note decreasing TB symptoms within days or weeks after starting medication will stop taking their drugs and will not complete their full treatment course, increasing the chance that their TB disease will reemerge and also contributing to the possible development of drug-resistant TB bacteria. In order to ensure completion of the treatment regimen, many—but not all—national TB programs use *directly observed therapy* (DOT), a system in which patients receiving TB treatment meet with a health worker or other trained person daily or at least several times weekly, either at a health clinic or in the patient's home or workplace. The DOT worker observes the patient taking the medicine(s) and is also available to discuss possible side effects and other challenges to adherence. TB treatment programs have also used incentives such as voucher programs—in which a patient receives a monetary or other benefit for completing treatment—to increase adherence to treatment regimens.[15]

While DOT and incentive programs are effective, they are time consuming and costly. Ensuring universal adherence to treatment regimens is virtually impossible for any disease, in any country—including in the United States—but the development of shorter TB treatment courses could result in higher treatment completion and cure rates while also saving time and money. Furthermore, high treatment-completion rates are also important in slowing the spread of drug-resistant TB.

---

[15] Institute of Medicine, *Ending Neglect*, 20.

4 | The Challenge of Drug-resistant TB

Over the last several decades, the emergence of drug-resistant TB has created significant challenges to the success of global TB-control programs.

TB drug resistance can develop when a patient's TB bacteria mutate after being exposed to small, but ineffective amounts of TB drugs—for example, when a patient fails to complete a full treatment course or only has sporadic access to medicine. The bacteria that survived that initial course of TB treatment are more likely to be at least partially resistant to one or more of the drugs being used. At that point, any drug(s) to which the bacteria have become resistant become ineffective for treating that person's TB disease. Only a few of these resistant bacteria need to survive for the patient to relapse with drug-resistant TB. By the same process, TB bacteria previously resistant to one or two TB drugs can evolve further to become resistant to even more TB drugs.

This evolutionary process has created a spectrum of TB drug resistance, from *mono-resistant TB* bacteria that are resistant to a single TB drug, to *multidrug-resistant TB* (MDR-TB) bacteria that are resistant to at least two of the most commonly used—and least expensive—TB drugs to *extensively drug-resistant TB* (XDR-TB) bacteria that are resistant to not only two or more "first-line" TB drugs, but also to at least two of the "second-line" alternative TB drugs that are kept in reserve to treat MDR-TB.[16]

In 2013, 136,000 MDR-TB cases were officially reported,[17] but estimates put the actual global MDR-TB caseload at 480,000, representing about 3.5 percent of all TB cases.[18] As a result, there were an estimated 210,000 MDR-TB deaths. Of particular concern is that of the 136,000 MDR-TB cases officially reported in 2013, only about 97,000 were started on appropriate "second-line" drug treatment, leaving 39,000 on treatment waiting lists, without adequate treatment, and thus able to continue spreading MDR-TB to others. Note that while this number of 97,000 on treatment represents 78 percent of officially reported MDR-TB cases, it represents only a small (20 percent) proportion of the estimated total MDR-TB caseload of 480,000.

Although overall global estimates of MDR-TB rates and numbers have been relatively stable, sharp increases in MDR-TB case numbers are being noted in some countries as testing for drug resistance becomes more easily available. Because TB drug resistance

---

[16] An even more extreme category of totally drug-resistant TB (TDR-TB) has been proposed, but the current consensus is that TDR-TB is not yet a distinct category. See World Health Organization, "'Totally Drug-Resistant' Tuberculosis: A WHO Consultation on the Diagnostic Definition and Treatment Options," March 22, 2012, http://www.who.int/tb/challenges/xdr/xdrconsultation/en/.

[17] More than half of these documented MDR-TB cases were found in only three countries: India, China, and Russia.

[18] World Health Organization, *Global Tuberculosis Report 2014*, 57.

usually evolves in individual patients, MDR-TB rates are higher in persons who had been treated previously for TB. However, an increasing proportion of drug-resistant TB cases are being reported in patients at the very outset of their first TB treatment course, at a time when the drug resistance could not have come about from inadequate prior drug treatment. This observation indicates that drug-resistant TB bacteria are increasingly being transmitted directly from patient to patient, an alarming development with the potential for a significant impact on future TB-control efforts.

Determining Drug Sensitivity of TB Bacteria

The rising prevalence of drug-resistant TB has serious implications for all aspects of TB control, particularly diagnosis and treatment. Because MDR-TB has been identified in an increasing number of locations, and because of the difficulties involved in its effective treatment, drug sensitivity testing (DST) is now recommended as a routine diagnostic procedure.[19] This change means that despite the small proportion of active TB cases with drug-resistant TB, the very possibility of drug resistance adds to the complication and cost of identifying and correctly treating all active TB cases. The specific drug-resistance patterns required for adequate treatment can only be identified using relatively expensive and time-consuming testing in sophisticated laboratories,[20] which are not available yet in many national TB programs. An inability to provide TB culture and drug sensitivity means that even experienced TB practitioners are "flying blind" in terms of their ability to provide the correct TB drugs. Efforts are underway to increase access of national TB programs to laboratories with DST capabilities.

Sputum culture remains the best method for determining TB drug resistance. The new molecular tests, such as GeneXpert, are useful for screening for the presence of TB drug resistance, but these tests *cannot* identify the specific drug resistance patterns that determine the best treatment options. The need to identify drug resistance as a routine component of TB diagnosis adds a challenging requirement to the wish list for a rapid diagnostic TB test, making efforts to develop such a test all the more difficult.

Treatment of Drug-resistant TB

The inability to use "first-line" TB drugs for MDR- and XDR-TB cases dramatically increases the costs and duration of treatment (12–24 months rather than 6–9 months).

---

[19] Ibid., 55.
[20] In order to correctly match each patient's TB treatment to the drug sensitivities of the TB bacteria infecting them, drug sensitivity testing must be done as a routine component of laboratory efforts to grow (culture) the TB bacteria.

Treatment success ("cure") rates are substantially lower—and death rates higher—among patients with MDR-TB and XDR-TB.[21]

Treatment and prophylaxis for MDR- and XDR-TB also results in more frequent and severe adverse effects from the alternative second-line drugs routinely used for treatment and for prevention.[22] A recent school-based MDR-TB outbreak provided a stark example of the need for better second-line drugs (Box 1).[23]

Notably, U.S. patients usually have access to more "second-line" MDR-TB drugs than patients in most low- and middle-income countries—allowing more leeway for drug regimen changes for adverse drug effects. Thus, adverse effects of second-line treatment in low- and middle-income countries may be even more severe and more difficult to manage, resulting in even lower treatment completion rates.

Box 1: Adverse Effects of Second-line TB Drugs

A teacher in California exposed 118 school children to multidrug-resistant TB disease. Of these children, 31 had positive TB skin tests indicative of TB infection and were recommended to have preventive therapy. Five parents refused preventive therapy for their children. Of the remaining 26 children placed on preventive therapy, only eight (31 percent) completed treatment with their originally prescribed drugs. The rest had to switch to alternative second-line drugs because they experienced severe side effects—including abdominal pain, vomiting, rash, joint and muscle pain, reddened eyes, photosensitivity, and signs of liver toxicity (the latter noted in blood tests). After the switch, another seven (27 percent) were able to complete treatment. However, even with access to these alternate drugs, 11 children (42 percent) were unable to complete preventive treatment for MDR-TB due to the severity of their adverse effects.

There is a great need to discover and develop additional options for treatment and prevention of MDR-TB and XDR-TB. And in fact, this specific research and development challenge is particularly time consuming and costly because TB treatment regimens for individual patients require the use of *combinations* of TB drugs to slow or forestall development of additional drug resistance. Because two drugs can potentially interact with each other and produce unintended interference or side effects, once a new *individual* drug is developed, additional research needs to be carried on out on each new *combination* of drugs.

Because an analogous set of challenges was faced successfully over the last 20 years in the development of current multidrug treatment regimens for HIV/AIDS (a process

---

[21] World Health Organization, *Global Tuberculosis Report 2014*, 54.
[22] Centers for Disease Control and Prevention, "The costly burden of drug-resistant TB in the U.S.," March 2014, http://www.cdc.gov/nchhstp/newsroom/docs/2014/MDR-XDR-Treatment-Infographic2014.pdf.
[23] Felice C. Adler-Shohet, Julie Low, Michael Carson et al., "Management of latent tuberculosis infection in child contacts of multi-drug resistant tuberculosis," *Pediatric Infectious Disease Journal* 33, no. 6 (2014): 664–6.

that has revolutionized the care of that previously untreatable infection), there is hope that similar attention to needed TB research programs can help address the challenges of MDR-TB.

5 | A Focus on Preventing TB Infection and TB Disease

Although effective *treatment* of people with active TB disease is a critical component of global TB control, the most important aspect of long-term reductions in global TB disease and mortality is *prevention* of transmission of TB infection to new human hosts. TB prevention involves two major components: *primary prevention of TB* is the prevention of the occurrence of initial TB infections; *secondary prevention of TB* is the prevention of the progression of latent TB infection to active TB disease.

Primary Prevention of TB Infection

There are three ways to halt the spread of TB infection.[24] First, rapid identification and effective treatment of people with known active (and contagious) TB can prevent TB infection in many of their previously uninfected family or other close contacts.[25] Second, the number of new TB infections can be reduced by minimizing the chances that those who are not yet infected with TB come into contact (e.g., within health care facilities) with people who have undiagnosed—and thus untreated—active TB. For example, people living with HIV (PLHIV) are a known high-risk group for TB coinfection, and many have not received TB testing or treatment (more on TB-HIV coinfection below). Therefore, clinics where HIV testing and counseling is done and/or where antiretroviral drugs are distributed are places where PLHIV without TB infection can come into contact with PLHIV who have undiagnosed and untreated TB disease. In addition to emphasizing the importance of TB screening and diagnosis in such settings, other measures that could be helpful include (1) improving ventilation in such facilities and (2) in clinics that handle both HIV and TB, separating known PLHIV from other patients arriving for TB diagnostic testing.

Finally, development and widespread use of an effective TB vaccine could significantly reduce or eliminate the chance of infection—even if recipients were exposed to people with active TB disease.[26]

---

[24] Infection control is one of the "three I's" that are recommended as routine components of global TB-control programs. Specific recommendations for implementing infection-control programs have been widely distributed.

[25] "Effective treatment" in this case refers to the correct drugs being provided and taken for the correct amount of time.

[26] Many research studies are currently underway to develop an effective TB vaccine. Many of these studies are focusing on improving the protection conferred by the existing BCG vaccine while an increasing number of studies are pursuing novel research designs. See World Health Organization, *Global Tuberculosis Report 2014*, 114–17; and Timothy Evans, "Preventive vaccines for tuberculosis," *Vaccine* 315 (2013): B223–26.

Secondary Prevention of TB Disease

Preventing latent TB infection from progressing to active TB disease requires two steps: (1) identifying people with latent TB infection and then (2) determining which of those should receive preventive treatment.

The most obvious approach involves screening people who are at particularly high risk for TB infection—such as people coming from or living in countries with high TB burden, PLHIV, close contacts of newly identified TB cases, or other vulnerable populations (discussed later)—to identify those already infected with TB. One specific version of this screening is called "contact investigation," in which persons identified as close contacts of known cases of active TB disease are screened by TB skin test (or blood test) to identify latent TB infection.

Once latent TB infection is diagnosed, patients can be provided with treatment for that infection with one of several regimens to significantly reduce the risk of progression of latent TB infection to active TB disease. Isoniazid hydrazide (INH) taken once daily as a single drug for six to nine months has been used for decades to treat latent TB infection, but fewer than half of patients given this regimen completed their treatment. U.S. TB programs are increasingly using two much shorter regimens that lead to much better completion rates. One regimen uses rifampin as a single drug taken daily for four months while the other uses isoniazid plus another newer medicine (rifapentine) taken once weekly for 12 weeks.[27]

TB-preventive therapy is also sometimes recommended for people without proven latent TB infection if they have recently been exposed to someone with known TB disease *and* if they are in one of the groups at higher risk of progressing from latent TB infection to active TB disease. Since TB drugs can have harmful side effects, the decision to provide preventative therapy should balance each individual's risk of developing active TB with his or her ability to complete the treatment and resource availability.

---

[27] Unfortunately, rifapentine is expensive and not easily available outside the United States.

6 | Complications of TB and TB-control Efforts

The global TB-control landscape is also complicated by additional challenges, including biological (TB/HIV coinfection, diabetes-TB comorbidity), population specific (pediatric TB, and TB in women and other vulnerable groups), and systemic (drug costs, lack of program accountability). These are each discussed briefly below.

Biological Complications of TB

HIV/AIDS

TB and HIV are epidemiologically and physiologically linked: in people infected with both, each disease increases the severity and accelerates the course of illness of the other. TB remains the single most common cause of death of PLHIV; at least 25 percent of the 1.5 million global AIDS deaths in 2013 were from tuberculosis.[28,29] Although the frequency of TB deaths is lower among PLHIV taking antiretroviral treatment (ART) for AIDS and although TB treatment success rates are higher in people taking ART, TB is still the most common infectious disease cause of death among that group. Conversely, about 25 percent of all TB deaths occurred in PLHIV. This two-way link highlights the urgency of prevention, screening, and treatment for TB among PLHIV.

The suppressed immune system caused by HIV infection is largely responsible for this large TB disease burden in coinfected people. Even those people with a current latent TB infection are at greater risk if HIV-infected; progression to active TB disease is 25–50 times more frequent in that group than in those people with latent TB infection who are not HIV-infected.

WHO has proposed the "Three I's" as an approach to TB/HIV coinfection: (1) Intensive case finding of people with active TB disease by regular and ongoing aggressive TB screening among PLHIV; (2) Improved TB infection control to prevent TB transmission in AIDS clinics and other sites where PLHIV congregate; and (3) Isoniazid (INH) drug treatment of PLHIV who have (presumed) latent TB infection to reduce their chances

---

[28] World Health Organization, *Global Tuberculosis Report 2014*, 83.

[29] Because TB is a disease that is often under-recognized based on clinical signs and symptoms, particularly in PLHIV, autopsy studies may provide a more precise estimate of TB's burden in patient groups. All four recent studies of patients dying with AIDS reported finding disseminated TB in at least 50 percent of autopsies. See Haileyesus Getahun, "Ongoing trials on empiric TB treatment for PLHIV: Prospects and challenges for policy recommendation" (paper presented at Conference on Retroviruses and Opportunistic Infections [CROI], Seattle, WA, February 24–26, 2015).

of developing active TB disease.[30, 31] The President's Emergency Plans for AIDS Relief (PEPFAR), U.S. Agency for International Development (USAID), and other U.S. programs support the emphasis on the "Three I's."

Two additional evidence-based "I's" have also been proposed to help address TB/HIV coinfection: (4) Integrated approach to TB/HIV coinfection by national TB and HIV programs and (5) Intensive use of antiretroviral drugs for PLHIV to reduce their risk of death from TB.

Recommendations have included HIV tests for new TB patients and regular TB screening for PLHIV. However, globally, fewer than half of new TB patients in 2013 had documented HIV test results, although numbers are rising slowly; 20 percent of these documented HIV tests were positive. (The corresponding HIV testing figures among new TB patients in the United States in 2013 were 88 percent tested and 7 percent HIV-positive.) Numbers of PLHIV routinely screened for TB globally are suboptimal and not yet considered reliable. Because TB disease and HIV disease each accelerate the course of the other and because available drugs can work to slow or arrest the progression of each of them, these gaps in TB and HIV testing represent a set of crucial missed opportunities in disease prevention.

Similarly, most of the world's 41 high-burden TB/HIV countries have not yet begun formal programs of providing isoniazid preventive therapy, representing another major missed opportunity to prevent the progression of latent TB infection to active TB disease.

A significant policy concern about TB/HIV coinfection is the potential long-term threat that TB represents to the life-saving successes of the PEPFAR program. In 2013, 78 percent of the world's HIV-infected TB cases were in sub-Saharan Africa and a large proportion of these cases were in PEPFAR's African focus countries where the bulk of PEPFAR's more than $50 billion has been invested. The U.S. government's 2010 Lantos-Hyde TB strategy clearly assigned the Office of the Global AIDS Coordinator—through PEPFAR—to be the lead agency for the U.S. government's response to global TB/HIV coinfection. However, PEPFAR only allocates approximately 3 percent of its resources to directly address TB issues. This matter is especially urgent given recent data about the frequency of coinfection in PEPFAR's African focus countries: the proportion of new TB patients who also have HIV infection ranges from the lows of 11 and 24 percent in Ethiopia and Côte d'Ivoire, respectively, to highs of 61, 62, and 62

---

[30] Intensive screening of PLHIV for TB is another of the recommended "Three I's" while isoniazid preventive therapy (IPT) is the third one. IPT is effective in those not infected with HIV as well as in PLHIV.

[31] World Health Organization, *WHO Policy on Collaborative TB/HIV Activities: Guidelines for National Programs and Stakeholders* (Geneva: WHO, 2012), http://www.who.int/tb/publications/2012/tb_hiv_policy_9789241503006/en/.

percent in Botswana, Zambia, and South Africa respectively.[32] Even higher numbers are seen in other African countries.

The challenges globally of addressing TB/HIV coinfection and codisease include: (1) achieving adequate coordination between TB and HIV programs at local, national, and international levels; (2) increasing the proportion of new TB patients who are tested for HIV infection; (3) increasing the proportion of PLHIV who are regularly screened for active TB disease; (4) increasing the proportion of PLHIV *without active TB disease* who are provided with isoniazid (or other) preventive therapy; (5) matching resource availability to current program needs; and (6) maintaining recent program gains during PEPFAR's complex program transition toward country ownership.

Without sufficient attention to addressing this set of TB/HIV coinfection issues, TB may continue to be a significant obstacle to PEPFAR's successes.

The Rising Challenge of Coexisting TB and Diabetes

Although the first link between TB and diabetes mellitus was recorded about 1,000 years ago,[33] diabetes continues to complicate TB-control efforts, and will likely exacerbate the problem as global diabetes rates are predicted to double over the next 15 years.[34]

Diabetes weakens the immune system, allowing the progression of latent TB infection into active TB disease. Patients with latent TB infection who also have diabetes are three times more likely to develop active TB disease than their nondiabetic counterparts and up to five times more likely to develop MDR-TB.[35]

To make matters worse, TB symptoms in people with both diseases differ from traditional TB symptoms; thus coexisting diabetes can complicate the identification and treatment of TB, resulting in either lower rates of case detection or misdiagnosis.[36] In addition, treating patients with coexisting TB and diabetes is more difficult; preliminary evidence shows that traditional TB and diabetes drugs such as rifampin and insulin, respectively, may counteract each other. In order to improve management of coexisting TB and diabetes, interactions between these and other TB and diabetes drugs need to be better understood.

---

[32] World Health Organization, *Global Tuberculosis Report 2014*, 85.

[33] International Union against Tuberculosis and Lung Disease and World Diabetes Foundation, *The Looming Co-epidemic of TB-Diabetes: A Call to Action* (Paris: The Union, 2014), http://www.theunion.org/what-we-do/publications/technical/the-looming-co-epidemic-of-tb-diabtetes.

[34] Currently, 172 million people have type II diabetes, and the number is projected to surge to 552 million in 2030. See Marcin Skowronski et al., "Tuberculosis and Diabetes Mellitus—An Underappreciated Association," *Archives of Medical Science* 10, no. 5 (2014): 1019–27.

[35] Ibid.

[36] Sara Bailey and Paul Grant, "'The Tubercular Diabetic': The Impact of Diabetes Mellitus on Tuberculosis and Its Threat to Global Tuberculosis Control," *Clinical Medicine* 11, no. 4 (2014): 344–47.

The global burden of coexisting TB and diabetes is likely to increase over the next few decades since diabetes rates are rising globally and approximately 80 percent of the future global diabetes burden is projected to be in developing countries,[37] where at least one-third of the population has latent TB. The confluence of these two diseases in countries with high burdens of both diseases will cause an increase globally in active TB disease over what might have been expected in the absence of diabetes. For example, recent studies from India, which accounts for 24 percent of the global TB burden, indicate that nearly half of all TB cases were found to have either diabetes or pre-diabetes associated with abnormal blood sugar levels.[38]

A greater understanding of coexisting TB and diabetes, including identification of better diagnostic methods and better treatment options, is necessary to prevent the growing global burden of diabetes from causing an analogous spike in TB disease.

Population-specific Complications of TB

Poverty

Tuberculosis is fundamentally a disease of poverty. It disproportionately affects the poor in part because of risk factors associated with poverty that increase susceptibility to TB: poor ventilation, overcrowded living and working conditions, and malnutrition.[39] In addition, impoverished TB patients often lack access to health-care facilities that can provide treatment and prevention options and may also be malnourished or coinfected with another disease. These components of poverty can delay patient diagnosis and care, and consequently facilitate the spread of disease.

TB also perpetuates poverty. Specific costs to patients and families include the direct costs of transportation, health care visits, diagnostic tests, hospitalization, treatment drugs, and other household expenses, in addition to the indirect costs of lost income and time. A study reviewing TB program data from eight African countries found that the average *pre-diagnosis* costs alone (transport, lost wages, testing, and clinic costs) totaled *catastrophic* levels—defined as more than 20 percent of average family income.[40] Another study of TB-related costs in Ghana, Vietnam, and the Dominican Republic found that the total direct and indirect costs were approximately equivalent to a year's income and that inability to work and other indirect costs far exceeded the direct costs of treatment and care.[41] The importance of these findings is that even if TB

---

[37] Ibid., 344.
[38] Skowronski et al., "Tuberculosis and Diabetes Mellitus," 1020.
[39] Approximately 95 percent of people who develop active TB disease are among the 4.4 billion people who live in developing countries, and almost a quarter of these are malnourished.
[40] K. N. Ukwaja et al., "The Economic Burden of Tuberculosis Care for Patients and Households in Africa: A Systematic Review," *International Journal of Tuberculosis Lung Disease* 16, no. 6 (2012): 733–39.
[41] V. Mauch et al., "Free Tuberculosis Diagnosis and Treatment Are Not Enough: Patient Cost Evidence from Three Continents," *International Journal of Tuberculosis Lung Disease* 17, no. 3 (2013): 381–87.

treatment costs were free (i.e., paid totally by the government), many families would still experience catastrophic costs.

Families of TB patients are often forced to take out loans or compel their children to support the family instead of attending school.[42] In addition, the cost of care may push patients to delay seeking care or stop their treatment early, which causes TB to spread, and in the latter situation, to potentially become drug-resistant. In cases where patients have MDR-TB, the direct and indirect costs are even higher, but the treatment success rates are lower.[43]

In sum, TB and poverty are in a well-documented cycle where one drives the other, and many current policy documents acknowledge poverty as a core determinant of health. While explicit poverty reduction goals are beyond the scope of most health programs, TB interventions must be planned with a clear understanding of the role poverty plays in the prevention, transmission, and treatment of TB.

Vulnerable Groups

There are other populations who, in addition to potentially being poor, are more susceptible to TB. Migrant workers, refugees, and other displaced people may be at greater risk because of crowding and because it is difficult to conduct effective contact tracing, diagnosis, and treatment of these migrating populations. They may also avoid or face discrimination from health care workers due to language and other cultural barriers. Homeless populations are also vulnerable for similar reasons.

Drug users are also at high risk of developing TB disease, at least in part because injecting drug use is also a primary method of HIV transmission, which can increase the risk of developing active TB disease.

The incarcerated population is another group vulnerable to TB. In some countries, prisons may account for up to 25 percent of a country's TB burden and, because crowding leads to more extensive spread of TB, prisoners may have TB disease rates that are 100 times greater than the nonincarcerated population. Prisons often lack the resources necessary to adequately screen and treat prisoners. Even if those processes are begun, continuity of care often cannot be ensured if prisoners are released prior to completing their treatment regimens.

The particular vulnerabilities of these and other specific populations need to be incorporated into local and national policies and programs for effective TB control.

---

[42] World Health Organization, "Eliminating the Financial Hardship of TB."
[43] A study in Peru demonstrated that nearly 40 percent of households affected with MDR-TB incurred catastrophic costs. See Tom Wingfield et al., "Defining catastrophic costs and comparing their importance for adverse tuberculosis outcome with multi-drug resistance: a prospective cohort study," *PLoS Medicine* 11, no. 7 (2014).

Pediatric TB

TB among children has been called a "hidden epidemic" in part because estimated numbers of pediatric TB cases are widely acknowledged to be undercounts. Reasons that many TB cases in children go unrecognized include, but are not limited to, (1) that children are often unable to produce sputum necessary for sputum microscopy and TB culture, making a confirmed TB diagnosis far more difficult than in adults[44]; (2) that many other childhood diseases mimic the signs of pediatric TB disease; and (3) that recommended family-centered TB contact tracing is often not done after adults are diagnosed with TB. For these and other reasons, the poor global control of childhood TB has been called "one of our biggest public health failures."[45]

A rough WHO estimate is that there were 550,000 new TB cases in children under 15 years old in 2013,[46] although other estimates are even higher.[47] Pediatric TB differs from adult TB in several important ways: (1) because of the immune system deficits associated with young age (infancy) and/or malnutrition, children with latent TB infection are more likely than are adults to progress to active TB disease; (2) although treatment of pediatric TB infection and disease is highly effective when the right drugs are provided in adequate doses, those drugs are often not available in liquid form in low- and middle-income countries; and (3) because they do not cough with as much force as adults, children with TB disease are much less likely to spread TB to others. In fact, most TB-infected children are infected by adult members of their own households.

In 2013, WHO, CDC, USAID, and others issued a *Roadmap for Childhood Tuberculosis*,[48] followed by a 10-module childhood TB training kit issued by WHO and the International Union against Tuberculosis and Lung Disease.[49] These products detail the effective and safe methods for preventing TB infection in children as well as for treating TB infection and disease, but a recent consensus of experts is that the technical knowledge and programmatic methods exist to successfully address pediatric TB at a global level but that "the motivation, means [resources], and coordination of services" are lacking.[50]

---

[44] Jeffrey R. Starke, "Improving tuberculosis care for children in high burden settings," *Pediatrics* 134 (2014): 655.

[45] Ibid.

[46] World Health Organization, *Global Tuberculosis Report 2014*, 14.

[47] Starke, "Improving tuberculosis care for children in high burden settings," 655.

[48] World Health Organization et al., *Roadmap for Childhood Tuberculosis: Towards Zero Deaths* (Geneva: WHO, 2013), http://apps.who.int/iris/bitstream/10665/89506/1/9789241506137_eng.pdf?ua=1.

[49] World Health Organization and International Union against Tuberculosis and Lung Disease, *Childhood TB Training Toolkit* (Geneva: WHO, 2014), http://www.who.int/tb/challenges/Child_TB_Training_toolkit_web.pdf.

[50] Starke, "Improving tuberculosis care for children in high burden settings," 655.

TB among Women

The approximate 3.3 million women with new TB disease in 2013 accounted for 37 percent of the estimated global total of 9 million cases and women comprised about 30 percent of the 1.5 million TB deaths during that year.[51] The reasons for this sizable male-female inequality are not fully understood, although it is notable that these gender differences in TB disease and mortality are not seen in PLHIV or in children.[52]

While biological differences in TB susceptibility have been noted and are continuing to be explored, the notable gender difference in TB notification and death rates may also be rooted in socioeconomic and cultural practices. One problem may be that women have lower case-detection rates due to their delaying care or their inability to access nondiscriminatory health facilities. In addition, women do not produce sputum samples as well as men, which might lead to lower detection, diagnosis, and treatment.

Even though women represent a smaller portion of TB cases, their central role in the household makes a focus on women particularly important. Once infected with TB, women of reproductive age progress from latent TB infection to active TB disease more frequently than men.[53] Any delay in seeking treatment for active TB disease can increase their risk of spreading TB to their children and other household members. In addition, TB-infected pregnant women are twice as likely as uninfected pregnant women to give birth to a premature or low-birth weight baby and four times more likely to die in childbirth.[54] HIV-infected pregnant women are at high risk of transmitting both TB and HIV to their infants.[55] These factors, plus that women are less likely to seek treatment than men, suggest that a focus on TB infection among women could have an outsized impact on the spread of TB.

Systemic Complications

Shortages of TB Drugs and Testing Materials

Shortages of both first- and second-line TB drugs have presented a problem in recent years throughout both the developing and developed world, including the United States. In addition to shortages of drugs, the material used for TB skin testing has also been in short supply.

---

[51] World Health Organization, *Global Tuberculosis Report 2014*, 14.

[52] Olivier Neyrolles and Luis Quitana-Murci, "Sexual Inequality in Tuberculosis," *PLoS Medicine* 6, no. 12 (2009).

[53] C. B. Holmes, H. Hausler, and P. Nunn, "A review of sex differences in the epidemiology of tuberculosis," *International Journal of Tuberculosis Lung Disease* 2, no. 2 (1998): 96–104.

[54] Action, "Tuberculosis: An Unchecked Killer of Women," fact sheet, 2011, http://www.action.org/resources/item/tuberculosis-an-unchecked-killer-of-women; and Janet Fleischman, *Tackling TB and HIV in Women: An Urgent Agenda* (Geneva: Global Coalition on Women and AIDS, July 2010), http://women4gf.org/wp-content/uploads/2013/10/Tackling-TB-and-HIV-in-Women-copy.pdf.

[55] Fleishman, *Tackling TB and HIV in Women*.

Reasons for these shortages are varied but include the limited number of manufacturers of these drugs (corresponding to the limited profit margins available), shortages of the raw materials used to manufacture the drugs, weak supply chains (including weak forecasting ability), and limited stockpiles.

The consequences of the intermittent shortages of drugs and testing materials include increasing development of drug-resistant TB (resulting in the need for prolonged and more expensive treatment and lower cure rates); prolonged periods of infectiousness in individuals who cannot access adequate treatment, which leads to more transmission of TB; inefficient use of staff time to seek out drug supplies; and increased treatment costs.[56]

Solutions have been proposed to alleviate shortages. Central stockpiling of drugs, sharing of drugs across countries, and market-shaping initiatives such as the Global Drug Facility (discussed in more detail below), have helped mitigate the problem. Research and development of new, cheaper drugs and testing materials are also essential to fixing this problem.

Program Costs

In addition to the biological and population-specific complexities of TB, the global TB-control effort is hampered by systemic shortcomings. One particularly problematic systemic failure is the cost of prevention and treatment. Approximately $8 billion is required to properly tackle the global TB epidemic in low- and middle-income countries, but there is currently a $2 billion funding gap (this does not include additional funding required for research and development of new vaccines, therapies, and diagnostics). According to WHO, 66 percent of the funding should go to detection and treatment of drug-susceptible TB; 20 percent for MDR-TB; 10 percent for rapid diagnostic tests and laboratory strengthening; and 5 percent for joint TB/HIV initiatives.

The *per patient* cost of treating TB varies by location and drug-resistance patterns. For drug-susceptible TB, the cost per patient in most high-burden countries ranged from $100–$500. Treating patients with MDR-TB ranged from $10,000 in low-income countries to $130,000 or more in higher-income countries like the United States.[57] As noted earlier, TB and poverty have a cyclic relationship to individual patients, which ultimately strains both domestic and international systems.

Evidence suggests that some national TB programs could benefit from revamping their overall approach to TB patients. For example, a recent South African study found

---

[56] Barbara J. Seaworth et al., "Interruptions in Supplies of Second-Line Antituberculosis Drugs—United States, 2005–2012," *Morbidity and Mortality Weekly Report* 62, no. 2 (January 18, 2013): 23–26, http://www.cdc.gov/mmwr/preview/mmwrhtml/mm6202a2.htm.
[57] Centers for Disease Control and Prevention, "The costly burden of drug-resistant TB in the U.S."

that reducing the hospitalization of TB patients (a practice no longer routine in the United States) could have a major impact of reducing TB treatment costs to both patients and national TB programs.[58]

The bottom line is that TB is highly expensive and debilitating, with the potential for catastrophic health and financial impacts for individuals, families, and health systems. Several aspects of TB treatment and prevention efforts could be improved in order to reduce costs and improve outcomes:

1. Better diagnostic tools would allow health workers to identify active (and therefore contagious) TB disease and begin appropriate treatment sooner.

2. Safer, better tolerated, and shorter treatment regimens—for both drug-sensitive and drug-resistant TB—will be required to improve completion rates, reducing the chances for reemergence, spread, and the development of resistance.

3. Access to additional second-line drugs with greater efficacy and fewer side effects could also help reduce the spread of drug resistance.

4. More family contact investigations, other screening for high-risk patients with latent TB infections, and targeted use of preventative treatment would reduce the number of patients who develop active TB disease.

Investment in any one or more of these efforts could have a major impact on the future success of TB-control efforts.

---

[58] Despite repeated studies indicating the lack of utility of hospitalization for most TB cases, the practice continues in some countries. See E. Sinanovic et al., "Impact of reduced hospitalization on the cost of treatment for drug-resistant tuberculosis in South Africa," *International Journal of Tuberculosis Lung Disease* 19, no. 2 (2015): 172–78.

7 | Institutional Actors on the Global Scene

Total funding for global TB prevention and treatment in 2014 reached approximately $6.3 billion, the vast majority of which (89 percent) came from domestic health budgets.[59] However, that domestic proportion varies greatly by country: domestic TB-control funding predominates in industrialized countries and other large economies, such as Russia and India, but international donor funding provides more than 90 percent of total TB funding in low-income countries with large TB burdens.[60] Essential actors in tackling global TB include a group of international organizations and other nongovernmental organizations such as the World Health Organization, the Stop TB Partnership, the Global Fund to Fight AIDS, Tuberculosis, and Malaria, and the International Union against Tuberculosis and Lung Disease, as well as several U.S. government agencies.

The Global Fund to Fight AIDS, Tuberculosis, and Malaria (Global Fund)

Established in 2002 as a public-private partnership, the Global Fund is the largest global donor of TB prevention and treatment resources. The Global Fund is a financing mechanism rather than an implementing agency, awarding resources to countries based on their expressed need(s) and on the technical merit of their grant proposals. A Country Coordinating Mechanism, the committee of national stakeholders required in each country by the Global Fund, both prepares funding proposals to the Global Fund and manages the resulting Global Fund awards. Since its inception, the Global Fund has distributed $4.7 billion in TB-specific awards, approximately 17 percent of its total disbursements.

The Global Fund's own policies are governed by an international board of directors that meets at least twice a year. In order to foster better in-country collaboration and optimize resources in countries with high burdens of both TB and HIV, in 2013 the Global Fund began requiring counties to submit joint TB/HIV program proposals.[61] While it is too soon to evaluate the outcome of this change, it is expected to have a positive impact on TB-control efforts in those countries.

---

[59] World Health Organization, *Global Tuberculosis Report 2014*, 92.
[60] Ibid., 100.
[61] Global Fund to Fight AIDS, Tuberculosis, and Malaria, *Joint Tuberculosis and HIV Programming: Information Note* (Geneva: Global Fund, April 2014).

The United States is the largest donor to the Global Fund, having provided $8.4 billion (31 percent) of the Fund's contributions through FY 2013. In FY 2014, the U.S contribution to the Global Fund was $1.65 billion, of which $295 million is used for TB prevention and treatment.[62] The FY 2015 U.S. contribution to the Global Fund is slated to be $1.35 billion, equivalent to $243 million for global TB programs.[63]

The World Health Organization's Global TB Programme

The Global TB Programme (GTB) of the World Health Organization is responsible for developing an overall global TB strategy and a series of evidence-based policies for TB treatment and prevention. GTB is also responsible for monitoring global numbers of TB cases, including MDR-TB cases, guiding the global TB research agenda, and coordinating technical assistance to countries with high burdens of TB, TB/HIV coinfection, or MDR-TB.

The WHO recently developed a *Post-2015 Global TB Strategy* designed to end the TB epidemic,[64] and it was approved by all 204 member states in 2014 (Box 2). It is based on three strategic pillars: integrated, patient-centered care and prevention; bold policies and supportive systems; and intensified research and innovation.

The WHO plays a critical role as a respected source for treatment guidelines, norms, and global disease monitoring. Unfortunately, it is woefully under-resourced, in part because of the recent economic downturn, as member states reduced their levels of support to WHO that resulted in a reduction in GTB's human and financial resources. Currently, the United States (through USAID) funds about 70 percent of GTB's total annual budget and provides additional technical support for development of new guidelines and policies.

---

[62] J. Stephen Morrison and Phillip Nieburg, *Strategic U.S. Leadership—Essential to Address the Global Tuberculosis Pandemic* (Washington, DC: CSIS, June 2014), http://csis.org/files/publication/140602_Morrison_StrategicUSLeadership_Web.pdf.
[63] The administration's Global Fund proposal for FY 2016 has been reduced to $1.0165 billion. See Adam Wexler and Allison Valentine, "The U.S. Global Health Budget: Analysis of the Fiscal Year 2016 Budget Request," Henry J. Kaiser Family Foundation, March 11, 2015, http://kff.org/global-health-policy/issue-brief/the-u-s-global-health-budget-analysis-of-the-fiscal-year-2016-budget-request/.
[64] World Health Organization, "The End TB Strategy," March 2015, http://who.int/tb/post2015_TBstrategy.pdf?ua=1.

Box 2: Abbreviated Version of the Post-2015 Global TB Strategy

Vision: A TB-free world, with zero TB deaths, disease, and suffering

Goal: End the global TB epidemic

2025 Milestones (v. 2015): 75% fewer TB deaths, 50% fewer TB cases; no families with catastrophic costs

Principles

1) Government stewardship and accountability;

2) Coalitions with civil society and communities;

3) Promotion of human rights, ethics, and equity;

4) Adaptation of strategy and targets at country level.

Pillars and Components

1) **Integrated patient-centered care and prevention**

   A. Early diagnosis, universal drug susceptibility testing, and systematic screening;

   B. Treatment of all with TB disease;

   C. Collaborative activities for TB/HIV and other comorbidities;

   D. Preventive treatment of persons at high risk.

2) **Bold policies and supportive systems**

   A. Political commitment and adequate resources;

   B. Engagement of communities, civil society, and public and private care providers;

   C. Universal health coverage, with vital registration, complete case notification and infection control;

   D. Social protection and poverty alleviation.

3) **Intensified research and innovation**

   A. Discovery, development and rapid uptake of new tools, interventions and strategies;

   B. Implementation research.

A complete version of the strategy is available at http://who.int/tb/post2015_TBstrategy.pdf?ua=1.

Stop TB Partnership

The Stop TB Partnership is composed of almost 1,200 international organizations, governments, academic institutions, private-sector groups, and nongovernmental organizations. It was established in 2001 after a series of high-profile global TB outbreaks increased awareness of the need for more effective TB-control activities.

The primary purpose of the Partnership has been to provide stakeholders with an open forum to express their viewpoints, an opportunity not always possible in other venues. Its 2011–2015 Global TB strategy has been praised for establishing meaningful, constructive goals for progress, including fostering sustained collaboration among partners; increasing political engagement by world leaders; promoting innovations in TB diagnosis and care; and ensuring universal access to quality-assured TB medicines and diagnostics.[65]

A crucial component of the Stop TB Partnership is its *Global Drug Facility* (GDF). The GDF is an innovative drug procurement mechanism that provides TB drugs to national TB programs at a reduced cost, thereby helping build a larger, more stable global TB drug market. The GDF also helps manufacturers to produce and provide second line (MDR-TB) drugs at a lower cost. It is now the largest global supplier of quality-assured TB drugs.

The United States has been involved in the Partnership since its inception. U.S. support includes a contribution, through USAID, to the budget of the Partnership itself, a large contribution to the GDF, and in-kind support through participation of U.S. government staff on the Partnership's coordinating board and on many of their various TB-related working groups.

International Union against Tuberculosis and Lung Disease (Union)

The Union is an international NGO based in Paris that works in more than 100 countries on issues affecting "lung health." Among its TB-related work, it provides technical assistance, organizes clinical and operational research, publishes a well-respected monthly journal, conducts training, and advocates for measures to advance global, national, and local TB control. Its annual conference is the largest global conference on control of tuberculosis infection and disease.

KNCV Tuberculosis Foundation

The KNCV Tuberculosis Foundation is a large Dutch NGO that focuses exclusively on the technical aspects of TB prevention and treatment. KNCV has been the principal partner with USAID's flagship global TB-control program over the last five years (FY 2010–2014). KNCV is also the principal recipient of USAID's newly awarded, five-year (2015–19), $525 million global "TB Challenge" program that, working with eight other NGOs, will focus on improving control of TB, including MDR-TB, through "effective, efficient and sustainable TB control strategies."[66]

---

[65] See Stop TB Partnership, *The Global Plan to Stop TB 2011–2015* (Geneva: WHO, 2010), http://stoptb.org/assets/documents/global/plan/TB_GlobalPlanToStopTB2011-2015.pdf.
[66] The name "KNCV" comes from the initials of the Dutch name for the foundation. See KNCV Tuberculosis Foundation, "Challenge TB," 2015, http://www.kncvtbc.org/challenge-tb.

Direct U.S. Government Support for Control of Global TB

The U.S. government has been involved in global TB-control activities for several decades. Until the late 1990s, the major U.S. role had been to provide technical assistance on TB prevention and treatment to countries through USAID and CDC. Since then, the U.S. role has expanded, and the United States is now the largest national donor to global TB-control efforts.

The U.S. government's current global TB strategy is based on the Lantos-Hyde Act of 2008,[67] a law that authorized up to $4 billion for global TB control during FY 2009–2013. The Lantos-Hyde Act also required U.S. agencies to develop a five-year global TB strategy that included support for international organizations such as WHO's Global TB Programme and the Stop TB Partnership.[68] Despite the ambitious goals set out in 2008, only about 30 percent ($1.2 billion) of the authorized amount was actually appropriated, and the shortfall has hampered the country's ability to fully implement its global TB strategy.

U.S. government resources addressing global TB-control issues are primarily provided through USAID; the Office of the U.S. Global AIDS Coordinator (OGAC), which manages PEPFAR; the Centers for Disease Control and Prevention (CDC); and the National Institutes of Health (NIH). Of these four, USAID has by far the largest global TB program and it plays a major role in all aspects of U.S. global TB activities. USAID has recently begun providing resources to "TB Challenge," its five-year (FY 2015–2019) $525 million flagship initiative to provide direct technical support to various countries' national TB programs, focusing on 27 priority countries. USAID is also the largest donor to the World Health Organization's Global TB Programme and to the Stop TB Partnership's Global Drug Facility.

Because of the growing importance of TB/HIV coinfection and codisease, OGAC, through PEPFAR, has continued use of some of its own resources to support the role of national TB programs in the integration of TB and HIV services.[69] For example, these funds can be used for HIV testing of TB patients, TB screening of PLHIV, prophylactic ARV treatment, counseling, and health system strengthening. However, OGAC allocates only about 3 percent of its total budget ($150–$160 million) to activities directly targeted at TB/HIV—despite TB being the most common cause of death among PLHIV.

---

[67] Tom Lantos and Henry J. Hyde United States Global Leadership Against HIV/AIDS, Tuberculosis, and Malaria Reauthorization Act of 2008, Public Law 110-293, 110th Congress, http://www.gpo.gov/fdsys/pkg/PLAW-110publ293/html/PLAW-110publ293.htm.
[68] U.S. Agency for International Development, *Lantos-Hyde United States Government Tuberculosis Strategy* (Washington, DC: USAID, March 2010), http://pdf.usaid.gov/pdf_docs/PDACP707.pdf.
[69] Recent amounts made available annually through this PEPFAR mechanism have been in the $150–$160 million range.

CDC is a major implementer of PEPFAR country programs, including those related to TB/HIV coinfection. CDC also works directly with partner ministries of health to strengthen surveillance systems, laboratories, and TB treatment programs and policies. CDC conducts patient-centered and program research to assess the value of promising new technologies for the management of adult and childhood TB and TB/HIV. Finally, under recently enacted global health security legislation,[70] CDC will also address MDR-TB in a limited number of countries.

The National Institutes of Health (NIH) is the single-largest funder of basic research on TB treatment and other global TB issues. It also focuses on translating the results of those basic research findings into the development of effective TB drugs and diagnostic tools.

---

[70] Jordan Tappero, "CDC joins hands with other USG agencies, WHO, Ministries of Health and other partners in the Global Health Security Agenda Launch," *CDC Updates from the Field*, issue 14 (Spring 2014), http://www.cdc.gov/globalhealth/healthprotection/fieldupdates/pdf/dghp-field-updates-2014-spring.pdf.

8 | TB in the United States Reflects the Global TB Burden

In 2013, 9,582 TB disease cases were reported in the United States, a 3.6 percent decrease from 2012 and a continuation of a slow but steady decline in case numbers that has occurred for 21 consecutive years.[71] Similar trends have been seen in U.S. TB deaths. In 2011, the most recent year with complete mortality data, there were 536 reported deaths from TB in the United States, a 67 percent decline from 1993.[72]

TB rates in the United States are significantly higher among people born outside the country. Although TB cases occurring in "foreign-born" persons are decreasing slowly and steadily, they are not decreasing as quickly as TB cases among native-born Americans. Consequently, the proportion of TB occurring in the foreign-born is increasing steadily and, in 2013, was 64.4 percent. The TB case rate of 15.6 cases per 100,000 foreign-born U.S. residents was 13 times greater than the rate of 1.2 cases per 100,000 among U.S.-born people.[73] In addition, foreign-born persons accounted for 88 percent of MDR-TB cases reported in the United States in 2013.

Overall, more than half of people with foreign-born TB in the United States in 2013 were born in one of five countries: Mexico, the Philippines, India, Vietnam, and China. In addition, 60 percent of foreign-born TB cases in the United States occurred in people who had been resident in this country at least five years.[74]

There is reasonable consensus among both U.S. and global TB experts that the U.S. goal of eliminating TB within its borders is not achievable without successfully addressing the issue of foreign-born TB. Research has suggested that investing in TB control in countries with moderate and high TB burden could not only reduce the toll of TB disease in the United States but could also be cost-effective, saving the United States $150 million over a 20-year period.[75]

---

[71] Brittany Moore et al., *Tackling Tuberculosis Abroad: The Key to TB Elimination in the United States* (Washington, DC: CSIS, June 2014), http://csis.org/files/publication/140604_Moore_TacklingTBAbroad_Web.pdf.

[72] Because of the need to obtain mortality data from death certificates provided by the various states' vital statistics office (rather than from state health departments), data on TB mortality necessarily lags a year or two behind data on TB disease occurrence.

[73] The TB case rate refers to the number of TB cases per unit of population, in this situation, cases per 100,000 people.

[74] Centers for Disease Control and Prevention, *Reported Tuberculosis in the United States, 2013* (Atlanta, GA: CDC, October 2014), Table 16, http://www.cdc.gov/tb/statistics/reports/2013/pdf/report2013.pdf.

[75] K. Schwartzman et al., "Domestic returns from investment in the control of tuberculosis in other countries," *New England Journal of Medicine* 353, no. 10 (2005): 1008–20.

The United States also faces TB drug shortages. This issue has been discussed extensively in the United States and potential solutions have been proposed: central stockpiling of drugs, sharing drugs across state lines, obtaining drugs (including those available within the U.S.-supported Global Drug Facility) from foreign manufacturers, improved forecasting of shortages to the U.S. Food and Drug Administration, and a centralized new drug application process to coordinate drug availability for patients.[76]

---

[76] Ibid.

9 | Overarching Challenges

TB is complex in its prevention, clinical presentation, diagnosis, treatment, and interactions with other illnesses. Although numbers of TB cases and deaths have been falling slowly both globally and in the United States, limited progress in TB's treatment and recent shifts in it epidemiology have created some concerns about its future magnitude and direction as a public health challenge.

When thinking about how to address global TB, U.S. policymakers need to keep a series of resource-related policy challenges in mind:

1. U.S. allocations for global TB treatment and prevention are not clearly matched to current and projected disease burdens and threats.

U.S. resources directed at global TB through USAID have recently been about 70 percent less than what was authorized by Congress in 2008.[77] Recent budget proposals from the current administration have suggested even lower numbers. However, "[TB] remains among the world's major killers of young adults . . . and saps strength and productivity from nations critical to improved global health and U.S. security."[78]

In the past, U.S. and other TB-control program budgets have sometimes been "consciously" reduced as case numbers fall, however slowly. However, TB is a chronic disease and the primary message from slowly falling TB case numbers is *not* that TB disease is going away. Rather, it is that most of the TB cases that are easiest to identify, diagnose, and cure have been taken care of and that a large proportion of the subsequent TB cases to be faced include TB cases that are likely to be the most difficult to find (e.g., TB cases in isolated rural populations), adequately treat, and render noncontagious. In addition, more complicated TB disease in the form of MDR-TB and TB/HIV codisease is just over the horizon. Finally, because of the clear linkages between domestic (U.S.) and global TB burdens,[79] policymakers should keep "enlightened self-interest" in mind as U.S. policy and decisions about allocating resources are being made about support for global TB-control activities.

2. A significant portion of TB cases go unreported—and in many cases undiagnosed and untreated—posing a major challenge to stopping the spread of disease.

---

[77] Note that resources directed specifically at TB/HIV coinfection are provided through PEPFAR. See Lantos-Hyde Act 2008.

[78] U.S. TB expert Gerald Friedland, as cited in Rabita Aziz, "TB Budget Cuts Proposed as U.S. Plans Improved Global Disease Responses," *Science Speaks: HIV & TB News* (2014).

[79] Moore et al., *Tackling Tuberculosis Abroad.*

Because people with active TB disease can easily spread the infection to others, the 3 million unreported—and, for many, untreated—cases pose a significant public health challenge. Improving access to diagnosis, treatment, and reporting of these missing cases would not only mean better outcomes for those 3 million people, but would also help stem the local and global spread of TB.

3. Future global patterns of TB disease are uncertain.

Although numbers of global TB cases and deaths have continued falling, albeit slowly, warning signs are on the horizon. Concern has been expressed recently that this ongoing decline in global TB numbers may be reaching a plateau.[80] A rapid increase in the number of global diabetes cases is predicted, which is likely to result in an increase in TB cases. Even more worrisome is the ongoing spread of MDR-TB from the cascade of patients (a) never being diagnosed, (b) not started on treatment, or (c) not successfully completing treatment. Thus, the numbers and complexity of future global TB cases may begin rising.

4. The remarkable successes of PEPFAR—and the growing numbers of PLHIV—need to be protected from the impact of TB, the current number-one killer of AIDS patients.

The TB disease burden among the growing numbers of PLHIV threatens the long-term integrity and success of PEPFAR, the United States' signature twenty-first-century global health initiative. The U.S. government has invested over $50 billion in PEPFAR since its launch in 2003 and currently supports life-saving antiretroviral treatment for an estimated 6.7 million people. Yet, as noted in a recent PEPFAR document,[81] TB remains the leading infectious disease killer of PLHIV and is particularly problematic among PLHIV in eastern and southern Africa, the areas that have received the bulk of U.S. HIV/AIDS funds.[82] Investment in more effective prevention and treatment of TB among PLHIV can help protect PEPFAR's extraordinary gains.

5. If not identified and treated with adequate preventive therapy, current latent TB infections will result in significant numbers of future active TB cases.

Focusing on treatment of TB disease without additional attention to controlling latent TB infection is repeating some of the conceptual errors made in the first 20 years of the AIDS pandemic, when attention was focused largely on people with AIDS, and less

---

[80] Anthony D. Harries, "Diabetes-tuberculosis Collaborative Activities: From Evidence to Action" (presentation at the 45th Union World Conference on Lung Health presentation at International Union against Tuberculosis and Lung Disease [IUTB] meeting, Barcelona, Spain, 2014), http://slideonline.eu/recordings/2014/14union/.

[81] President's Emergency Plan for AIDS Relief, "Technical considerations," Office of Global Aids Coordinator, 2015.

[82] Adapted and updated from Morrison and Nieburg, *Strategic U.S. Leadership—Essential to Address the Global Tuberculosis Pandemic.*

on those people with early HIV infection who had not yet progressed to AIDS. In that scenario, the numbers of people dying fell rapidly only after large numbers of HIV-infected people began receiving treatment prior to developing clinical AIDS symptoms.

Globally, 2 billion people are estimated to have latent TB infections and the estimated number of latent TB infections in the United States is 11 million. Although many, if not most, people with latent TB infection have a low risk of progressing to active TB disease, among other smaller subpopulations (e.g., people with HIV infection or diabetes) the risks are much higher. Using currently available risk profiles and relatively simple and inexpensive interventions such as TB preventive therapy to prevent the onset of active and contagious TB is a necessary step to arresting the spread of this disease.

6. TB in the United States increasingly reflects the global TB burden.

Most tuberculosis disease occurring in the United States in recent years is being identified in U.S. residents who were born in other countries. [83] Although the numbers of such foreign-born TB cases are decreasing slowly, U.S. TB-elimination goals originally established in 1989 are unlikely to be achieved without significant U.S. TB-control investments in countries with high and moderate TB burdens, especially in those countries that are major sources of foreign-born U.S. TB cases.[84]

---

[83] Moore et al., *Tackling Tuberculosis Abroad*, 2.
[84] Ibid., 8.

10 | Closing Comment

Global tuberculosis is an exceedingly complex infection and disease, both on its own and in its interactions with cultural, genetic, economic, disease, and other factors. Beyond an understanding of the disease's causes and transmissibility, the formulation of adequate policies, the mobilization of adequate resources, and implementation of robust programs to control global TB will require a clear understanding of the enormous disease and economic consequences of TB and of the knowledge and resource gaps in our current approaches.

| Appendix A. TB Testing and Diagnosis

Table 1. Some Methods for Initial Testing (Screening) to Identify Tuberculosis Infection

Screening Test	Description	Advantages	Disadvantages
TB Skin Test	TB test fluid injected under skin; site examined for redness /swelling in 48–72 hours	Point-of-care Low cost Widely available*	Frequent false positives in those who had BCG vaccine Requires care in injection placement Care needed in examining site at 48–72 hours
TB Blood Test (e.g., IGRA*)	Identifies immune system response to TB infection	Specific for TB infection Not reactive after BCG	Higher cost Requires sending blood serum to lab Not widely available in low- and moderate-income countries
Chest X-ray	Provides evidence of lung TB	Low cost Widely available	Can detect other diseases Not specific for TB Does not identify *latent* TB infection
Four-Question History	Asks about recent TB symptoms: fever, night sweats, chronic ($\geq$3 weeks) cough, weight loss	Low cost Point-of-care Limited training needs	Does not identify latent TB infection Can be positive in other diseases Most useful in those with high TB risk (e.g., PLHIV)

*Interferon gamma release assay, such as Quantiferon™.

Table 2. Some Methods for Definitive Diagnosis of Tuberculosis Infection

Diagnostic Test	Description	Advantages	Disadvantages
Sputum Smear	Search under microscope for TB bacteria in phlegm	Point-of-care Low cost Reliable with skilled user	A few other bacterial types appear as TB Requires skilled user
Urine Test	Measures level of chemical from TB bacterial cell wall ("normal" level = 0)	Point-of-care Easier to obtain urine than sputum Very specific if positive Rapid (<1 hour)	Sensitivity may be less than sputum smear Accuracy is still being investigated
Sputum Culture	Detects TB bacterial growth	Unequivocal proof of TB "Gold standard" in TB diagnosis Allows drug-sensitivity test	Requires sophisticated laboratory Not widely available* Results may require 6–8 weeks
Rapid Molecular Tests	Detects TB (bacterial) DNA in sputum	Highly specific	Requires sophisticated laboratory Not widely available*
GeneXpert	One type of rapid molecular testing	Rapid results Specific for TB and one type of drug resistance	Costly (machine, infrastructure, cartridges) Requires dedicated machine operator Requires stable power supply Not widely available*

*Many low- and middle-income countries do not have this laboratory capacity.

Table 3. Differences between Latent TB Infection (LTBI) and Active TB Disease[85]

Someone with Latent TB Infection	Someone with Active TB Disease
Does not feel sick	Usually feels sick
Has no symptoms of TB infection	TB disease symptoms can include: chronic cough ($\geq$3 weeks), coughing up blood, fever, weight loss, chills, night sweats, fatigue, chest pain
Cannot spread TB to others	*Can* spread TB to others
Usually has positive TB skin test and/or TB blood test	Usually has a positive TB skin test and/or TB blood test
Has a normal chest X-ray	May have an abnormal chest X-ray
Has *negative* sputum smear and laboratory culture	May have a *positive* sputum smear and culture
Should probably receive LTBI treatment to reduce chance of developing active TB disease	Needs treatment for active TB disease
Is one of as many as 2 billion people with latent TB in the world	Is one of approximately 9 million new cases of TB disease globally per year

---

[85] Adapted from Centers for Disease Control and Prevention, *Questions and Answers about Tuberculosis, 2014* (Atlanta, GA: CDC, 2014), http://www.cdc.gov/tb/publications/faqs/pdfs/qa.pdf.

| Appendix B. Additional TB Resources

Global TB

- World Health Organization, *Global Tuberculosis Report, 2014* (Geneva: WHO, October 2014), http://apps.who.int/iris/bitstream/10665/137094/1/ 9789241564809_eng.pdf?ua=1.

- Stop TB Partnership, *The Global Plan to Stop TB 2011–2015* (Geneva: WHO, October 2010), http://www.stoptb.org/assets/documents/global/plan/ TB_GlobalPlanToStopTB2011-2015.pdf.

- Stop TB Partnership website: http://www.stoptb.org/.

- U.S. Agency for International Development (USAID) tuberculosis website: http://www.usaid.gov/what-we-do/global-health/tuberculosis.

- Centers for Disease Control and Prevention, "Global Tuberculosis (TB)," 2014, http://www.cdc.gov/tb/topic/globaltb/default.htm.

- Thomas R. Frieden, Karen F. Brudney, and Anthony D. Harries, "Global Tuberculosis: Perspectives, Prospects and Priorities," *Journal of the American Medical Association*, no. 312, October 2014, 1393–94.

Domestic (U.S.) TB

- Centers for Disease Control and Prevention, *Reported Tuberculosis in the United States, 2013* (Atlanta, GA: CDC, October 2014), http://www.cdc.gov/tb/statistics/ reports/2013/pdf/report2013.pdf.

- National Tuberculosis Controllers Association website: http://www.tbcontrollers.org/.

- Stop TB-USA website: http://stoptbusa.org/.

- Curry International Tuberculosis Center website: http://www.nationaltbcenter.ucsf.edu/.

- Lawrence Geiter (ed.), *Ending Neglect: The elimination of tuberculosis in the United States* (Washington, DC: National Academy Press, 2000).

- State-specific TB data are available from each state's TB-control office. For state-specific contact information, see the list at http://www.cdc.gov/tb/links/tboffices.htm.

| Appendix C. Abbreviations and Glossary

ART: Antiretroviral treatment, a drug or drugs given to persons living with HIV/AIDS.

BCG: Bacille Calmétte-Guérin vaccine, a hundred-year-old TB vaccine that provides only weak protection against TB for children and essentially no consistent protection for adults; BCG is sometimes given to infants in countries where TB is common. BCG can result in false-positive TB skin tests, complicating the diagnosis, treatment, and reporting of actual TB infections.

Case: A specific instance of disease occurrence

CDC: Centers for Disease Control and Prevention, an agency of the U.S. Department of Health and Human Services that is charged with funding and managing national programs to control diseases of public health importance

Contact: Person who has been exposed to TB infection from someone with TB disease

Disease surveillance: Collection, analysis, and use (for policymaking) of specific data on the numbers and characteristics of cases of disease occurring in a population

DOT: Directly observed therapy, where a healthcare worker meets with a TB patient daily or several times a week to watch medications being taken, thereby ensuring completion of the TB treatment regimen.

DR-TB: Drug-resistant tuberculosis, consisting of TB bacteria that are resistant to one or more of the currently available TB treatment drugs; see MDR-TB (below)

Drug susceptibility test: Laboratory test that measures growth of specific TB bacteria over time to determine whether these TB strains are susceptible or resistant to specific TB drugs.

DST: Drug sensitivity testing, the laboratory-based identification of drug sensitivity and drug resistance of specific strains of TB bacteria that are infecting specific TB patients.

Elimination of tuberculosis (TB elimination): Reduction in the annual case rate of tuberculosis to <1 active case/100,000 population

FDA: Food and Drug Administration, an agency of the U.S. Department of Health and Human Service that, among other things, is responsible for ensuring the safety and efficacy of medications used in the United States.

GDF: Global Drug Facility, created in 2001, is the world's largest public-sector provider of first-line and second-line drugs to national TB programs.

GTB: Global Tuberculosis Programme is the office within the World Health Organization that provides global leadership on a wide range of critical TB-control issues, including policy recommendations for—and provision of technical support to—national TB programs, monitoring global TB burdens, and helping set the global TB research agenda.

IGRA: Interferon gamma release assay, a blood test to identify the presence of TB infection

Infection: Situation in which TB bacteria (or other organisms) have entered the body in a way sufficient cause an immune response.

Incidence (of disease): Occurrence of new disease within a fixed time period, for example, one year. See "prevalence of disease" (below).

INH: Isoniazid hydrazide (usually just called *isoniazid*), one of four medicines often used to treat TB disease.

IPT: Isoniazid (INH) preventive therapy, an oral anti-TB regimen that reduces the chance of latent TB infection progressing to active TB disease.

LMIC: Low- and middle-income countries.

LTBI: Latent tuberculosis infection, where the TB bacteria are walled off and effectively inactivated, but still alive in the human body.

MDR-TB: Multi Drug-resistant Tuberculosis, a more extreme type of TB drug resistance in which the TB bacteria are resistant to two or more of the most commonly used, safest, and least-expensive TB drugs.

NIH: National Institutes of Health.

OGAC: Office of the Global AIDS Coordinator, an office within the U.S. Department of State that manages the President's Emergency Plan for AIDS Relief (PEPFAR). The current U.S. Global AIDS Coordinator is Ambassador Deborah Birx, M.D.

PEPFAR: President's Emergency Plan for AIDS Relief, a U.S. government initiative that has provided more than $50 billion to heavily affected countries since 2004 to help prevent, treat, and mitigate the impact of HIV/AIDS.

PLHIV: People living with HIV (infection), that is, HIV-positive people

Prevalence of disease: Refers to the cumulative number of cases of a specific disease that are present in a particular population at any given time. Prevalence differs from a related concept, *incidence* of disease, which refers to the number of *new* cases that develop in a given period of time.

"Second-line" drugs for TB: These drugs are specifically intended for the treatment of drug-resistant TB and are different from the "first-line" drugs usually used to treat drug-sensitive TB. In general, second-line drugs are less effective, more expensive, have more side effects, and require longer treatment regimens than the drugs used for drug-sensitive TB. Some of these second-line drugs have been in short supply globally.

Surveillance: See "disease surveillance" above.

TST: Tuberculin skin test (TST), used to identify those people who have been infected by/with TB bacteria.

Two-step tuberculin testing: A baseline procedure consisting of a second TST procedure two to three weeks after the first one to help clarify whether a "positive" TST response is due to a "boosted" response to the first TST versus a new TB infection.

USAID: United States Agency for International Development, the U.S. government's external development agency.

XDR-TB: Extensively drug-resistant tuberculosis, a rare strain of bacteria is resistant to nearly all medications used to treat TB.

WHO: World Health Organization, the health component of the United Nations.

| About the Authors

Dr. Phillip Nieburg is a board-certified pediatrician with additional formal training completed in infectious disease (two-year fellowship), preventive medicine (two-year residency), and public health (MPH program) and with service as a U.S. military physician. From 1977 to 2003, Dr. Nieburg served as a medical epidemiologist in various programs at the Centers for Disease Control and Prevention (CDC). His CDC work involved research, program monitoring and teaching in various domestic and global health fields such as vaccine-preventable diseases, famine and refugee relief, child malnutrition, HIV/AIDS, and tuberculosis. He has worked extensively with various UN and other international agencies and with other U.S. government agencies. Since 2003, Dr. Nieburg has been a senior associate with Center for Strategic and International Studies (CSIS), initially working with its HIV/AIDS Task Force and since 2008 with its Global Health Policy Center. His major interests there have included aspects of HIV prevention, maternal mortality prevention and the collection and use of outcome and impact data to evaluate global health programs. He also works as a consultant with Project HOPE (Millwood, VA) and Akeso Associates (Seattle. WA) and is a visiting associate professor in the Department of Pediatrics at the University of Virginia (Charlottesville).

Talia Dubovi is deputy director and senior fellow with the Global Health Policy Center at the Center for Strategic and International Studies (CSIS). Prior to joining CSIS, she spent six years on Capitol Hill, most recently as appropriations associate/counsel for Representative Nita Lowey (D-NY), where she covered a wide range of foreign affairs issues and supported the representative in her work as ranking member of the Appropriations Subcommittee on State, Foreign Operations, and Related Programs. Ms. Dubovi also served as counsel to the House Oversight Subcommittee on National Security and Foreign Affairs and previously worked on human rights and judiciary issues for Senator Richard Durbin (D-IL). Before working in Congress, she was an associate at Latham & Watkins LLP and a fellow with Human Rights Watch's Refugee Program. Ms. Dubovi is a member of the Board of Directors and cochair of the American Planning Board of Humanity In Action, an international nonprofit organization that works for the protection of the rights of minorities. She is also a fellow with the Truman National Security Project. She holds a B.A. from Amherst College and a J.D. from the University of Michigan Law School.

Sahil Angelo is program coordinator and research assistant for the Global Health Policy Center at CSIS, where he conducts policy research focusing on infectious diseases, health systems strengthening, and global health security. He is also responsible for program planning, outreach, and administrative support. Prior to joining CSIS, he worked with Partners In Health. He graduated from Boston College, cum laude, with a B.S. in biology and international studies, with a focus on global health.